THE I CAN'T CHEW COOKBOOK

By

JEAN BLY

Contents

Legal Notes

INTRODUCTION

Hello, my name is Jean. I had dental implant surgery in my bottom jaw and stitches on the gum line and was not able to use my lower dentures for at least five weeks. This meant a liquid diet or very soft foods. Upon my release from the hospital, the dietitian handed me the only menu she could find to fit my need for liquids or soft diet. She confirmed soup, mashed potatoes and baby food would be my only options.

Thinking I had to east these few items for several weeks to a few months left my mind racing. Using a little imagination, I felt I could do better than that. I know there are elderly people who need a few ideas other than soup or baby food. There are those who have only a few teeth or not teeth at all. My jaws do not go together when my dentures are not in my mouth, this makes it difficult to chew. Now, being able to have only my upper dentures in was a challenge as to what I could eat.

Here, then, are a few ideas. Remember what your dentist has set for you when you are fixing your meals. Being able to use my tongue and only my top dentures, I had to think of what I could easily work in my mouth and be palatable at the same time. Your situation will dictate what you can tolerate.

Taking smaller bites and working the piece of food in your mouth will give you a satisfied feeling as chewing does. Concentrate on the food and the feeling of not chewing will soon pass. Remember you can overeat when food is easy to eat.

Upon finishing a meal, I rinsed my mouth out with warm salt water. This cleaned any small particles from the stitches I had in my gums. This is a good idea if you have had an extraction; do this carefully. These recipes and ideas are great when your stitches are out and your dentist recommends a diet of soft food until your healing is complete. With implants, this can take as long as six months. Baby food or soup only would be very boring.

Remember you are eating differently, so your bowel movements will differ. Your body will adjust in a short time and will be back to normal. A laxative should not be necessary.

Patience is the key to good eating and keeping healthy while your healing is taking place.

The following recipes and ideas are with my husband, Bruce, and I found could give me variety as well as nourishment. Some of them are every day fare that we often don't think of. Some of them are to put your imagination to work and come up with what you like. Mix and match any combination that you feel will benefit your situation and palate. You will not feel deprived and your healing time will pass much easier.

When the brand name is mentioned, I am not endorsing or recommending that specific product, it simply was the I chose to use and is mentioned as a guide for you.

Happy eating. Soon you, too, will say NUTS TO SOUP ONLY.

Jean Bly

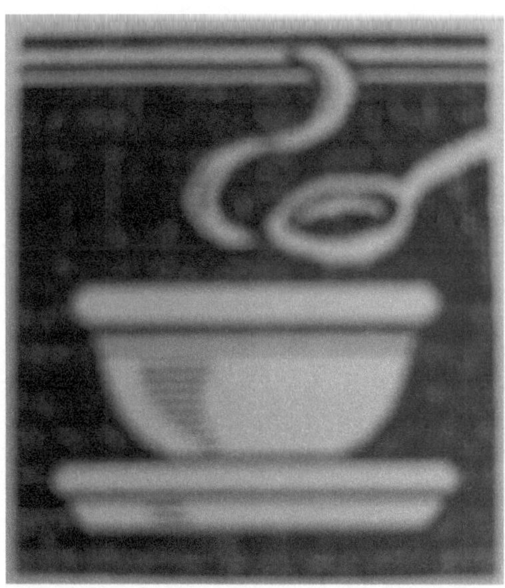

THE I-CAN'T-CHEW

COOKBOOK

BEVERAGES

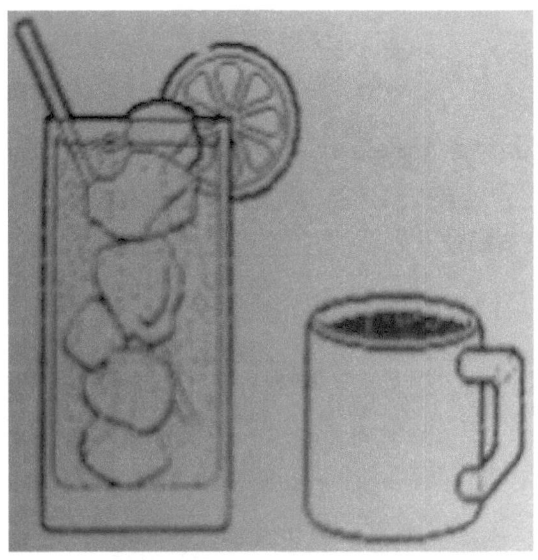

DIET OR REGULAR POP

I found that while I was talking antibiotics, the diet drinks did not taste very good. I used regular pop during this time. When my medication was no longer needed, the taste returned to normal.

BOUILLON, CHICKEN OR BEEF

This was very good the first couple of days after surgery when you don't know what you want. If you are on a salt restricted diet this is not a good choice. I could not tolerate the low sodium type. I would rather do without.

LIPTON SUGAR-FREE FLAVORED ICE TEA

HERBAL TEA

HOT COCOA MIX

I used the type that uses water not milk.

COFFEE, REGULAR/DECAF

FRUIT/TOMATO JUICE

Check to see if the acid in the tomato juice will affect your medication before drinking. Dr Dye says to watch "acidic" drinks as they can also cause nausea/vomiting, especially important to avoid postsurgery. Watch caffeine in cocoa or coffee, it is a stimulant. DON'T DRINK ALCOHOLIC BEVERAGES WITH MEDICATIONS.

BREADS AND BAKED GOODS

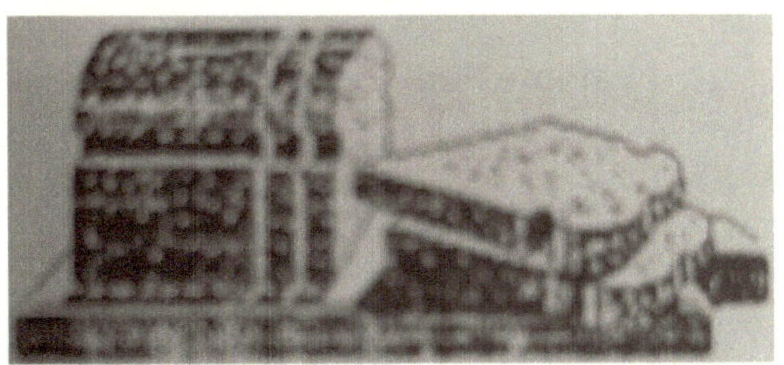

SWEETHEART LITE WHITE BREAD

Using Sweetheart LITE enriched bread was my choice. It has more natural fiber than whole wheat bread. It has only forty calories per slice. It contains natural vegetable fiber only…with no alpha cellulose (which is derived from wood pulp), a common ingredient in other reduced-calorie breads. This and other information can be found on the wrapper of the Lite bread. I found It a good choice because it crumbles in your mouth, and this makes it easier to eat.

PANCAKES

Use the mix of your choice or make homemade. Remember not to overcook or over brown, this makes them hard to eat and you want to be able to mash them with a fork. This, of course, will change if you are able to use both upper and lower dentures or the healing of your mouth permits. They are still an enjoyable soft food.

BISCUITS

I found that my homemade biscuits were easier to eat than the ready-made dairy type. This is the recipe I use.

Biscuits
- 2 cups sifted flour
- 4 or 5 tbsps. Shortening
- 3 tsps. baking power
- 2/3 (about) cup of sweet milk or buttermilk
- 3/4 tsp. salt
- 1 tsp. sugar

Sift dry ingredients together and cut the shortening in with a fork or pastry cutter; the ingredients should be cold. Add the liquid to the flour, just enough so the dough is light, soft, but stiff enough to handle. Put the dough on a floured board and mold it lightly into a ball, handling as little as possible. Roll very gently to ½-inch thickness and cut with glass dipped in flour or with 2-inch cutter. Place on greased pan. Pre-heat oven to 450 degrees F. and bake 12 to 15 minutes. Serves 4 to 6. I love these with white milk gravy. This really makes them east to eat. Yum.

HARDEE'S CINNAMON & RAISON BISQUITS

I love these biscuits (my husband does not like them). Not being able to take a bite, having only top dentures, I still was able to eat them easily. I was a mess and covered with frosting when I was finished, but it was well worth it.

P.S. When I could have my lower dentures in, I made just as big a mess as before. Perhaps I'm just sloppy.

CAKE

All types without nuts are good. To use with a sauce, I used angelfood cake. Cake is a food that is easy to eat so don't eat too much, the calories and fat count can really add up.

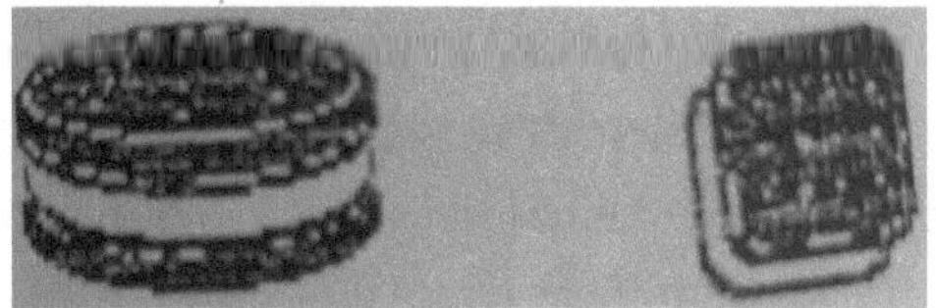

COOKIES

The ones filled with frosting are good. Sugar cookies are a good choice, too. Any cookies that don't have nuts or large chunks can be dunked and swallowed with ease. Don't overdo these as they are loaded with fat and calories.

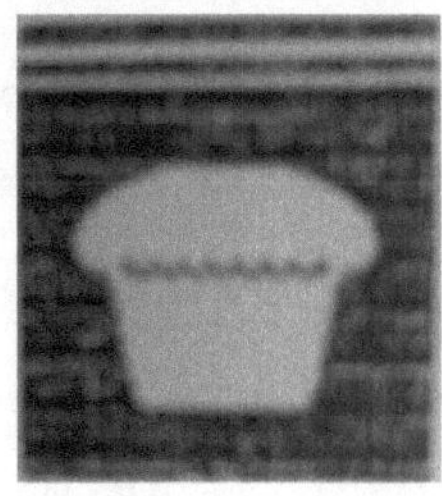

MUFFINS

I used the store bought type as they were more crumbly than homemade. You will find when the food crumbles it does not feel like you have a mouth full of glue.

PIE

Just about any kind can be eaten as long as there are no nuts or any texture that is considered a hard food. Cream pies are wonderful. Don't undo all your hard work by eating something that is putting pressure on your jaws and gums.

POP TART-TYPE PASTRIES

These are flaky enough to eat when put in a toaster. The Strudel type pastries were a little tough to chew without both upper and lower teeth. Your preference may be different, they may be more to your liking.

My stitches were removed sixteen days following surgery. Time will vary with each person and type of implant. I was not to use my bottom denture until five weeks had passed. I was surprised to find when I finally put in my lower teeth, I had trouble chewing. I had done very well without my teeth. The gum line was tender and after that length of time, it felt like I had a real mouthful.

Much to my surprise, I could not eat bacon, but you can bet I will try bacon again and again until I can eat at least one piece. I think I missed bacon more than any other food. Raisins and nuts had to be cooked in something in order to eat them without hurting my mouth. I didn't push the nut eating because that was putting undue pressure on the tender gums. I want my implants to heal as quickly as they can. It will be sometime yet before I can eat everything as before, but the care I take now will pay off when I can eat normally with my new dentures attached to my implants.

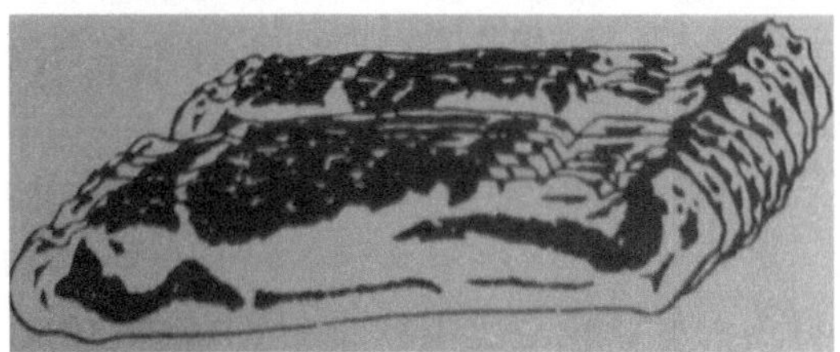

Cereals/Grains/Pasta

Cream of Wheat

Instant Quaker Oatmeal

I found the Blueberry type hard to swallow.

Quick Cooking Oatmeal

Zoom

Putting brown sugar in hot cereals while cooking is a nice flavor enhancer. Use a substitute sweetener if you prefer, it is good either way. Remember your mouth is tender, so let the cereal cool a little bit. I used 2% milk in order to cut out some of the fat and calories. Cold cereal had to set in order to get soft enough to eat. I did not like it, but if you like soggy cereal, it might be all right for you. If you have teeth, of course, you can eat dry cereal with ease. If you are healing from implant surgery, use a little caution with cereal with nuts. It is best to avoid raisins.

Quick Grits

Use as a cereal, serve with gravy or eat as a side dish with eggs.

Cous-cous

This is a Moroccan Pasta, quick to fix and very easy
to eat, with or without teeth. I even put spaghetti
sauce on it, it was really good used this way.

Pasta is not easy to eat when you have stitches, or
with few or no teeth. I found that Cous-cous was a
nice alternative at these times. Orzo, an enriched
macaroni product, is also a nice change, and it is also
good with a sauce. Use both products in place of rice
or potatoes. When you are not feeling your best, a
change in your diet is nice. We often get stuck in a
rut with our meals.

Macaroni & Cheese Dinner

Fast to fix and a good choice. The macaroni is small
enough to eat with little trouble. I cooked it a little
longer for a softer texture.

Rice

Rice is very versatile and can be eaten like a cereal,
in puddings as a dessert, steamed or fried. It is also
good with soy sauce or with gravy. We like it fried.

HAM FRIED RICE

Ham Fried Rice
- 2 tblsps. Olive oil or your choice of oil
- ½ medium onion, chopped
- 2 eggs beaten (optional)
- 3 cups steamed rice
- 1 cup cooked ham, diced
- 3 small strips red or green pepper, chopped, or use ¼ cup green peas.

In large frying pan, heat 1 tblsp.oil to hot, pour eggs in pan, stir to set, and remove from pan. Add rest of oil. Lightly brown onion, pepper, and diced ham. Stir in the rice. I like to heat the rice for 2 minutes in the microwave before putting it in the pan. Stir to mix, add egg, separating as you stir. Season to taste.

This is a meal by itself. I could not eat this with the ham or any type of meat until I could use both top and lower dentures. Beef, lamb, or any meat of your choice goes very well in fried rice. It is good meatless, I then use about a cup of cooked mixed vegetables.

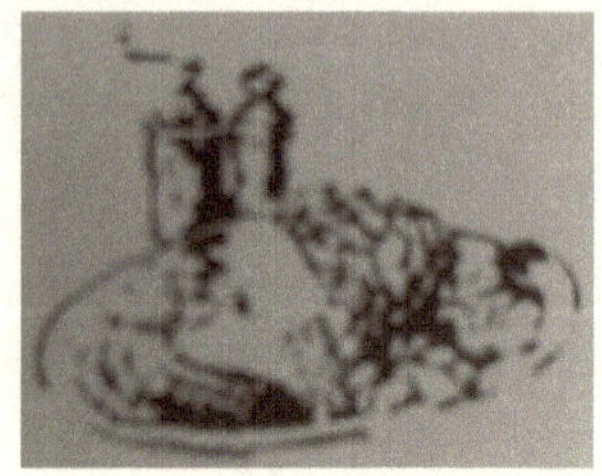

Dairy Products

Be sure to use lowfat products in order to cut down on fat grams. Compare the fat grams and calorie count on the product you choose.

Creamed Cottage Cheese

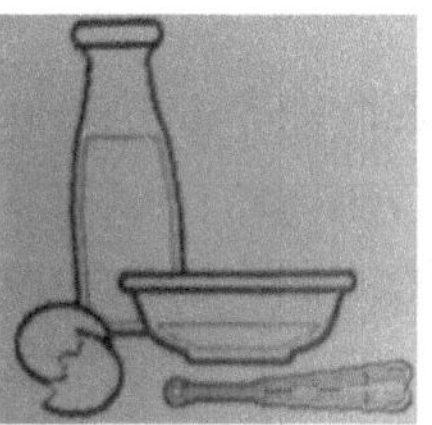

Lowfat Ice Cream/Ice Milk

Use the flavors without nuts or pieces of candy.

Lowfat Milk

I used 2% milk (skim milk seems like water)

Touch of Butter Spread

This spread is one of the lowest in fat grams.

Lowfat Yogurt

The fat content varies widely among different brands. Most of the fruit in the yogurt was in small pieces which made it easy to swallow.

Velvetta-Type Cheese product

This is a soft enough cheese that it will almost melt in your mouth. It is good in sandwiches and is great melted and placed over your favorite vegetables. Use only once in a great while, as with all cheese products.

When our son was in high school, it seemed like he lived on toasted cheese sandwiches. I found if I toasted the sandwich lightly and dunked it in tomato soup, I could have a toasted cheese sandwich. It was wonderful.

Cheese Spread

Another soft and easy-to-use product.

Frozen Milky Way Ice Cream Bars

These are not lowfat but are wonderful with or without teeth as an ego booster, or if you have the need to feel sinful.

Frozen Fudgesicles

If you have a need for chocolate, this is a good choice.

Eggs

Eggs are very easy to fix and eat, use according to your diet guidelines. I found it was easy to overuse eggs. Here are a few ways I used eggs.

Soft Scrambled Eggs

Soft Scrambled Eggs
- 2 eggs
- 1 tblsp. Water
- salt & pepper to taste

Use spray for pan, heat to hot, pout beaten eggs into pan. Using fork, move continually until eggs are soft set. Cooking too long will make them harder to move in your mouth.

Topping these on occasion with Picante Sauce was a real nice change.

POACHED EGG ON TOAST

Poached Egg on Toast
Bring water to boil in small saucepan, add 1 tsp
vinegar to water, this holds the egg in shape so it
doesn't spread all over the pan. Break eggs in
separate bowl, then slip one at a time into the boiling
water. Turn down heat to simmer, cook at low
simmer until set. Carefully remove with slotted spoon,
place on one or two pieces of Lite toast, dot with
butter or margarine, season with salt and pepper.

POACHED EGG WITH MILK TOAST

Poached Egg with Milk Toast
- 1 egg, poached (in milk, about 1 cup)
- 1 piece of Lite white bread, toasted very light
- 1 tblsp. Grated cheese (optional)

Bring milk to low boil, turn heat to low simmer. Slip
eggs one at a time into simmering milk, poach egg to
soft set. Remove carefully with slotted spoon. Place
toast in soup bowl, sprinkle with the cheese, carefully
place poached egg on toast, pour milk over all, dot
with butter, season to taste. Delicious. This is great
for an evening meal as well as for breakfast.

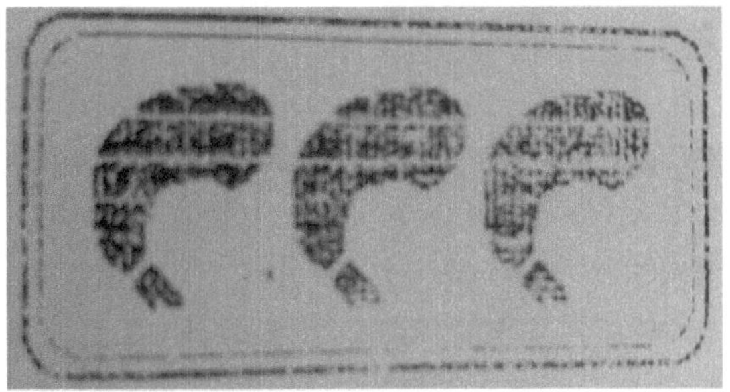

Scrambled Eggs and Tiny Shrimp

Scrambled Eggs and Tiny Shrimp
- 6 eggs, beaten
- 1 can tiny shrimp (drained & rinsed)
- 1 tblsp. Water
- salt & pepper to taste

Beat eggs with water. Spray pan with low calorie spray, heat to hot, pour in eggs, cook to soft set, add shrimp. Remove from heat, do not overcook, season to taste. This will serve 2-3 people. I serve it with thin sliced tomatoes. A nice treat for an evening meal.

SOFT-BOILED EGGS WITH TOAST

Soft-Boiled Eggs with Toast
- 2 cups boiling water
- 2 eggs in the shell
- 1 or 2 slices lightly toasted bread
- salt & pepper to taste

Bring water to boil in saucepan, lower eggs into water with spoon, set timer for 4 minutes. Run eggs quickly under cold water in order to handle, yet not cool egg too much. Crack egg in half with knife, use teaspoon to remove egg from shell, season to taste, a dot of butter is nice. Use toast to dunk in eggs.

FRUITS/DESSERTS

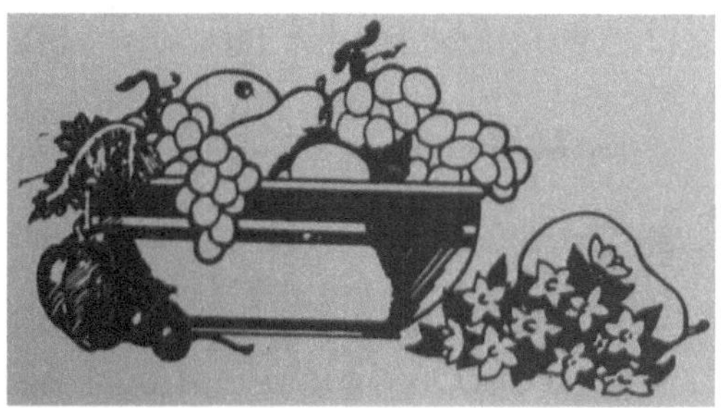

APPLES

I found if I cut the apple in small pieces and cooked it in the microwave until it was tender, I could eat the peeling, which provided some fiber. Eat your favorite apple. I choose Royal Gala. My daughter Ivy lives in Yakima Washington, and she was able to send them to me by the boxful.

APPLESAUCE BLENDER STYLE

Applesauce Blender Style
- 1 apple (your choice)
- 1 tsp. brown sugar
- cinnamon (as much as you like)

Cut apple in small pieces, leave the peeling on, put in microwaveable bowl. Microwave for about 2 minutes. Let cool until warm. Put in blender, pulse until fairly smooth.

This is wonderful on vanilla ice cream or great as is.

BANANAS

These are a naturally wonderful eating fruit, teeth or
no teeth.

PEACHES

Place a peach in boiling water for 1 minute. Remove
carefully with slotted spoon. Run under cold water
and remove the skin. If you have teeth, eat out of
hand. If you don't have teeth, remove pit cut in pieces,
and microwave until tender enough to eat. For a
souce, put in the blender and pulse until smooth (put
in sweetener if you like). Add cinnamon. Enjoy!

PEARS

This fruit I buy when it is quite ripe. Peel and eat as
is, if you can, or slice and cook until tender and serve
with chocolate sauce for a real treat.

STRAWBERRIES

Wash and eat as they are, or slice and put in the
blender, pulse one or two times, and add sweetener
of your choice. Serve over angelfood cake or ice
cream. A great fruit.

TOMATOES

I have a hard time thinking of a tomato as a fruit, but it is. I used them when they were quite ripe.

Remove the skin by putting in boiling water for one or two minutes, remove carefully with slotted spoon, run under cool water in order to handle, peel and slice. I cut the light colored center out which was a little hard, this made them much easier to eat.

I bought Picante Sauce. This was also very good on eggs.

WATERMELON

Many people like watermelon, I dislike all types of melon. It is very low in calories and can be eaten like it is when sliced. My husband says it is delicious, if you like melon this is a good choice of fruit.

There are many kinds of fruit so try the ones of your choice. Experiment with them, it's fun.

PUDDINGS

Any of the instant or cooked are good. Pistachio pudding was not easy eating, it was better when I had my lower dentures in. I often put a dollop of lowfat whipped topping on the pudding.

JELLO

All flavors of these are good and light after a meal. I
use the sugar free, then I have only 8 calories, and
can use a light topping.

Any of the baked goods already mentioned in that
section.

MEATS/POULTRY/FISH

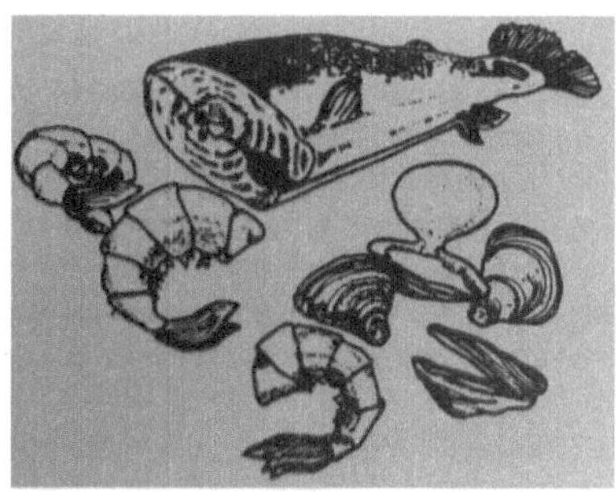

Meat is the hardest of all food to be able to eat. If you have your own teeth, or very good dentures, you are lucky.

Having loose dentures before and now healing from the implant surgery, I have not been able to really eat meat for some time. I am eagerly awaiting the healing of my mouth in order to have the abutments on my new implants for my dentures installed, then I can enjoy a piece of meat.

Thanks to my husband's concern he tried many ways to fix meat in order that I might eat a somewhat normal diet. Without a solid set of teeth and without the pain that accompanies loose dentures, this was not an easy task. The following steak recipe is a favorite of ours and can be enjoyed by anyone.

I am putting it first as it was the first steak I could eat. Thanks, Bruce.

Steak à la Bruce

Steak à la Bruce
- 2 medium venison or beef steaks about ½ inch thick
- 12 soda crackers (crush to very fine crumbs)
- 2 eggs (beaten with ½ egg shell of water)
- flour seasoned with salt and pepper

On a solid bread board, cut steak in 3 to 4 pieces each, pound each piece with meat mallet vey well to tenderize. Have crumbs, flour, and eggs in separate bowls big enough to place the meat in, in order to coat. Dip each piece first in flour, then in egg mixture, then in crumb mixture, shake off excess. Lay on paper towel to set coating while you heat oil for frying. Have oil in pan to a depth in order to deep fry steak, about 350 degrees. Carefully slip one steak at a time in the hot oil, cook only about 3 at a time. Cook each until nice golden brown, drain and place on plate covered with paper towel. Repeat until all steak is cooked. These are tender enough to cut with a fork and are wonderful to eat.

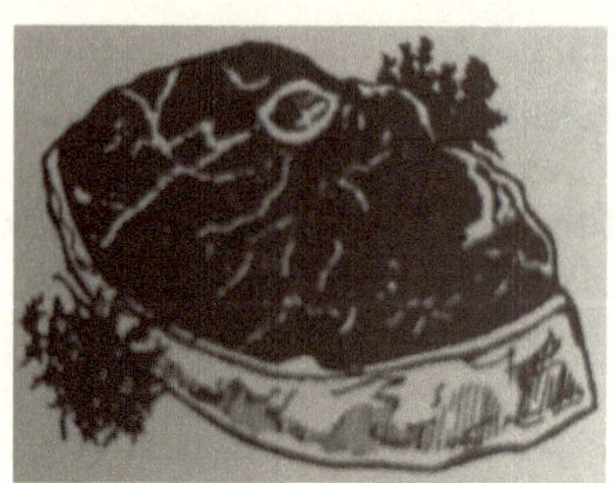

SLOPPY JOES

Sloppy Joes
- 1 lb. ground beef.
- 1 jar Sloppy Joe mix
- hamburger buns or Lite bread

In frying pan on low heat, use a fork to break up the ground beef. Continue using fork until you have fine pieces of beef, cook until done but not brown. If it is in large pieces or is brown, it is hard to eat. Pour in sauce and heat through. Serve on buns or bread. Even with no teeth these can be eaten quite easily. If you have teeth you can brown the meat and leave pieces larger. Remember I only had my top denture and tongue to use so I cooked what was easy for me to eat.

TAMALES

Use your choice of canned tamales. I place the can in the refrigerator until cold so I could remove some of the fat from the gravy before I heated them. Open the can and place tamales, with paper on in the saucepan, remove fat that has hardened in gravy. Heat very slowly, without adding extra liquid. Place tamale on plate, remove paper, be careful the will be hot. Mash with fork, mix in gravy.

Leave whole for those with teeth. These are really good. I served them with a carrot pattie and steamed broccoli. This made a nice meal.

HAMBURGER GOULASH

Hamburger Goulash
- 1 lb. ground beef
- 1 medium onion, diced
- ½ green pepper (optional), diced
- 1 tblsp. Parsley, dried or fresh (chopped up if fresh)
- 1 jar spaghetti sauce (or homemade)
- ½ of 1 lb. package pasta (shape of your choice)

Bring water to a boil, add 1 tsp. salt and pasta, cook until tender, drain. While pasta is cooking, spray frying pan with spray, break up and lightly brown ground beef with diced onion, green pepper. Add sauce and heat thoroughly. Mix beef mixture with pasta, sprinkle with parsley. While I had stitches in my mouth, I put this in the blender and pulsed only until the pasta was in small pieces. It may not look all that good but it sure beat eating baby food. Of course, leave as is for the rest of the family to enjoy.

Hamburger or Sausage Gravy

Hamburger or Sausage Gravy
- 1 lb. ground beef or sausage
- 3 tblsps. flour
- milk, approximately 3 cups

Brown beef or sausage, add flour to meat, cook to incorporate flour, don't brown, add milk slowly, stirring constantly. Gravy will start to thicken. The amount of milk will vary, start with three cups, as gravy thickens you will adjust accordingly and add more milk if gravy is too thick. Turn heat to low cook for about five more minutes. Season with salt and pepper to taste. Serve on homemade biscuits or on Lite bread. Good eating.

CORNED BEEF SUPREME

Corned Beef Supreme
- 1 can corned beef
- 1 medium onion, diced
- 1 egg (beaten)
- dry mustard

Heat frying pan, add a small amount of oil or use spray for pan. Cut or break up corned beef in pieces, put in mixing bowl with diced onion, beaten egg, mix well. Pour into frying pan, turn heat to low, let cook to brown underneath side. Carefully place plate large enough to cover pan on pan, hold plate and carefully flip meat out on plate, slip meat back in the pan and brown the other side. Sprinkle lightly with dry mustard. Remove from pan, serve hot.

VENISON OR BEEF STEW

Venison or Beef Stew
- 2 tblsps. butter flavored shortning
- 2 lbsps. good quality stew meat (remove any fat)
- 1 small onion, diced
- 1 medium carrot, diced
- 1 large potato, cut in large cubes
- 3 ripe tomatoes, peeled and chopped, or 1 small can
- 1 small bay leaf
- 1 tsp. salt
- ¼ tsp. pepper

In medium saucepan brown meat in shortening on high heat. Add bayleaf, salt and pepper, add water to cover meat. Boil for one hour, check often and add water as often as needed to cover meat. Add tomatoes, turn heat to low, cook covered an additional hour. Turn heat to medium, add potato, cook until tender. Serve. This is a meal in a bowl. I cooked it this way and it was tender enough for me to eat, yet was together enough for my husband to enjoy.

BAKED SWISS STEAK

Baked Swiss Steak
- 1 ½ lbs. beef round or chuck steak about 1 inch think
- ¼ cup flour
- 2 tsps. salt
- ¼ tsp. pepper
- 2 tblsps. beef drippings or shortening
- 1 clove garlic, finely chopped
- 2 cups onion, sliced thin
- 2 cups stewed tomatoes (1 can)
- ½ cup tomato juice
- ½ cup celery, diced
- 1 tsp. Worchestershire sauce
- 3 drops hot sauce

Cut beef in 4 oz. pieces, or leave in one place. Combine flour, salt, and pepper and pound into both sides of beef. Saute garlic and onions in beef drippings. Remove onions from pan, set aside to use later. Brown beef on both sides. Put in backing pan, and onions and other ingredients. Cover and bake in slow oven (300 degees F.) two or three hours or until meat is tender, or simmer on top of stove. Remove lid during last part of cooking to thicken sauce. Preparing steaks the day before they are to be served saves time and lets the tomatoes have a tenderizing action on the meat.

We found cooking a day ahead and reheating brings
out even more flavor. These steaks are excellent and
are good enough for company or a family treat. Very
easy on the tender mouth.

CHICKEN AND DUMPLINGS

Chicken and Dumplings
- 1 fryer, cut up
- 1 med. onion, cut in pieces
- 1 small carrot, diced
- 1 small stalk of celery
- 1 tsp. poultry seasoning
- chicken bouillon cube (optional)
- salt and black pepper to taste

Put all ingredients in large saucepan. Cover with
water. Bring to boil, turn heat down to simmer,
cook for one hour. Remove chicken with a slotted
spoon to plate to cool. Remove meat from bones.
Return meat to pan. Heat to boiling. Meanwhile
make dumplings.

Dumplings

Dumplings
- 1 cup flour
- ½ tsp. salt
- 3 tsps. baking powder
- 1 egg
- 1/3 cup milk

Sift dry ingredients together, beat egg and milk, mix together to a soft dough. Drop by spoonful in chicken and broth. Cover with lid and simmer for about fifteen minutes. Do not lift the lid to look or the dumplings will fall. These can be put in any broth.

I found boiled chicken, when hot, east to eat even when I had no teeth. With teeth it is great cold and can be eaten in sandwiches or as is in the chicken and dumplings.

FOIL-BAKED FISH

Foil-Baked Fish

- 4 fish fillets (1 pound)
- 2 tblsps. sliced green onion
- 1 cup sliced mushrooms
- ¼ tsp. thyme
- 1/8 tsp. salt
- 1 medium-size apple, sliced
- 1/8 tsp. ground black pepper
- 1 packet Butter Buds made into liquid, or pat of regular butter

Preheat oven to 350 degrees F. On four separate pieces of aluminum foil, arrange fish fillet with ¼ cup mushrooms and a few apple slices. Combine Butter Buds, onion, thyme, salt and pepper and pour over fish. If using butter, just place a pat on each fillet. Wrap up each serving tightly, sealing ends well. Bake about 15 to 20 minutes or until fish flake easily. This recipe is found in Cooking for the Health of It. It fit my need for soft food so I included it hear for you to enjoy. This is easy to fix for the whole family. You have more calories with butter. Fish, baked, panfried or steamed is ideal to eat anytime, not just when you have mouth problems.

Pork and Beans

Pork and Beans

Canned was my choice. They were easy to eat besides being nourishing. However, I yearned for potato salad when I ate them, while I had stitches in my mouth. As soon as I could have my lower dentures in, I promptly made the potato salad.

I found roasting meat was not a wise choice as far as easy eating. Boiling meat or using the pressure cooker turned out to be the best choice for me. I am hoping this all will change when my implants and my new dentures are in place. Roasting meat was a fine choice when I had teeth to chew it with.

Bruce did not seem to suffer at all during our trials and errors, as he could eat whatever we prepared.

Soup

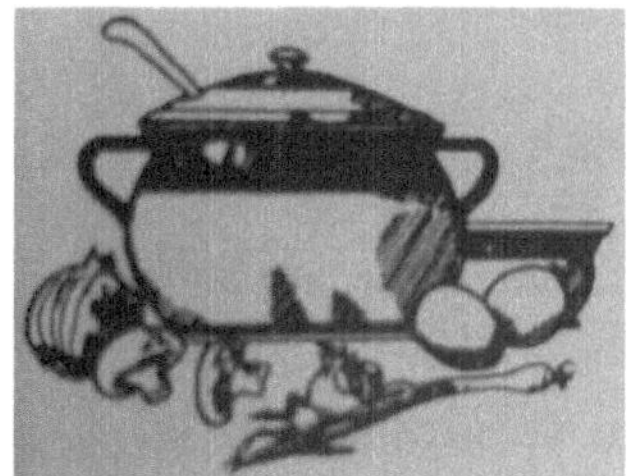

The varieties of soup are endless, so I certainly did not discount it. I chose to eat a variety of other foods which, hopefully, have given you a few ideas in this book.

Bruce made his famous potato soup which is a family favorite. He diced the bacon very small so I could eat it. I have included it here, maybe you will have it as a favorite of yours.

Potato Soup and Riblets

Potato Soup w/Riblets
- 2 medium potatos, diced
- 1 medium onion, diced
- 1 small stalk celery, diced
- 2 to 3 slices bacon, diced very small
- 2 cups milk
- salt and pepper (to taste)

Place potatoes, onion, celery and bacon in medium saucepan, add water to just cover ingredients. Boil until potatoes are tender (about

10 minutes). Do not drain, add milk to pan with water, check for seasoning.

The amount of salt will depend on the saltiness of the bacon. Heat to the boil, drop riblets by small spoonfuls in hot liquid. Turn heat to low, simmer for about 20 minutes covered. Riblets are not as tender as a dumpling, they have more substance to them. Don't peek.

RIBLETS

Riblets
- 2 to 3 eggs
- ½ tsp. salt
- ¼ tsp. pepper
- flour

Beat eggs, salt and pepper, add flour enough to make thick batter, not enough to be dry, but think enough to drop liquid by the spoonfuls.

I could not eat the riblets without my teeth, but savored the small bits of bacon. This is a delicious soup with or without the riblets.

CHILI

Canned or homemade chili is very good, if you have a tender mouth don't use the hot variety.

VEGETABLES

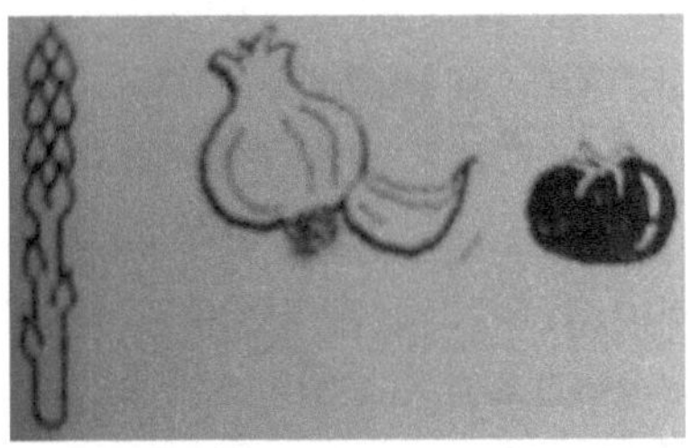

Vegetables are so easy to use and good to eat, whatever shape our mouth or teeth are in. Without my lower dentures, I put them in the blender but left some bulk to them, not smooth like baby food. Unlike President Bush, I love broccoli and ate it quit often. Blend a few times to find your preference in texture. I also found you have to cook the vegetables a little longer than you normally would. I still found them to be very good and enjoyable to eat. This was one instance when I steamed the vegetables different for Bruce than for myself.

CARROT PATTIES

Carrot Patties

- 4 to 6 medium carrots, cut in small rounds, cooked
- 2 tblsps. onion, finely minced
- 1 egg
- 6 soda crackers (approximately)
- season to taste
- small amount of shortening (for frying)

Cover carrots with water, boil until very tender.
Mash carrots as you would mash potatoes. Add
finely minced onion and egg, mix well. Crush
crackers and add a few at a time to mixture. This
will not be a stiff mixture. Heat skillet to medium,
add shortening, and with spoon ad enough carrot
mixture to make small patties, keeping heat low
enough not to brown very much.

Remember, you can't eat these if there is a hard
crust on them when you have stitches, no teeth or
you mouth is tender for surgery. If you do not
have any mouth problems they are great when
nicely browned. Potato patties can be make the
same way, just omit the carrots.

CAULIFLOWER

I steamed this a little longer than you would
normally so I did not have to use the blender. It
was easy to eat and seasoned with a little butter,
salt and pepper. If you like to use a dip, it would
be good for this also.

GREEN BEANS

Eating canned green beans was easier to eat than fresh cooked or frozen green beans. They had to be cooked a long time in order to be tender enough to eat. This is an idea for a change in the normal heat and eat bean especially if you like and miss bacon.

JEANS BEANS

Jeans Beans
- 1 can green beans, with liquid
- 1 tblsp. minced onion
- 1 tblsp. red pepper, chopped
- 2 slices bacon, fried and crumbled
- salt and pepper to taste

Put all the ingredients in a small saucepan, bring to boil. Season to taste.

CREAMED ONIONS

Creamed Onions
- 2 large onions, diced
- ¼ cup milk
- 1 tblsp. cornstarch
- 1 tsp. butter or margarine (optional)
- salt and pepper to taste

Place diced onion in medium saucepan, add water just to cover onions. Cook until tender, do not drain. Mix milk and cornstarch, add to water and onion mixture, cook and stir until thickened. If too thick, add more milk. Season with butter, salt and pepper. This is good as a side dish or is great on a baked potato.

POTATOES

Whether you boil, bake or fry and lightly brown potatoes they are wonderful. Use them often. Remember it is what you put on them that is fattening, not the potatoes.

DRY BEANS

Cooked in your favorite way makes a nourishing meal and takes the place of meat. The canned variety are quick and easy to use.

THE I-CAN'T-CHEW COOKBOOK is not by any
means a complete cookbook and was not ment to be.
My goal was to share with you what I learned and
tried during this time when eating is hard and very
boring. I hope you will try at least one idea and recipe
in order to make your healing time pass in a more
pleasant way. Having the support of my husband and
my dentist, Dr. Timmon Dye, and his wonderful staff,
and good food have been a great help. If you have a
great mouth and perfect teeth I hope you will try a
recipe or two also. Your meals do not have to be
boring or soup only. Be creative, and happy eating.

P.S. Seven weeks after my surgery, I had a piece of
bacon. Yes, it was great, but not easy to eat.

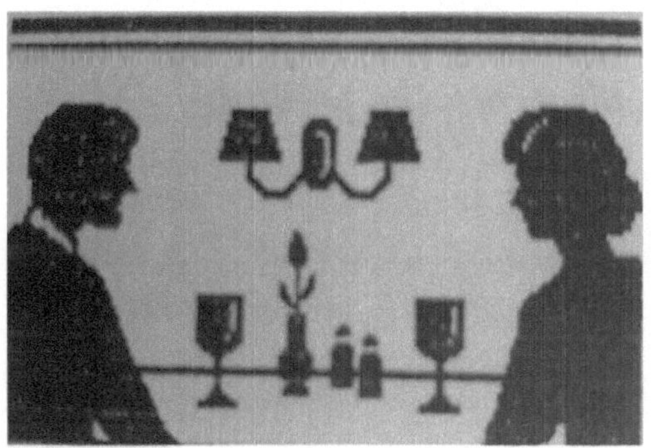

INDEX TO RECIPES

ABOUT THE AUTHOR

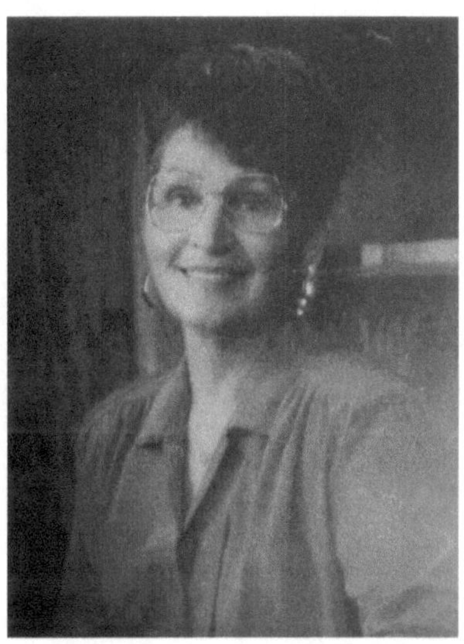

AUTHOR NAME is Jean Bly

Jean Bly was born in Craig, Colorado. She and her husband, Bruno, have been married for over twenty-two years, and they have six children.

With the children all grown, Mr. and Mrs. Bly now reside in the quiet of the mountains of Montana.

Mrs. Bly received her Associates of Arts degree from Eastern Montana College recently, in Applied Psychology, and she is looking forward to working in the human services area. Mr. Bly is retired from the United States Air Force and spinning sheep's wool into yarn for Roundup Wools. This is the author's first published book.

Original Hardbound Edition ISBN 0-8062-4791-6

A Hearthstone Book

Carlton Press, Inc. New York, N.Y.

Find out more at Book and Author Page

Or visit Bly House Media

BOOKS BY BLY HOUSE MEDIA.

THE I-CAN'T-CHEW COOKBOOK was a partial inspiration; we also publish children's books (soon).

Our goal was to publish Jean Bly's book as close to the original as possible. We used a new iphone to take pictures of the original clipart used in the original hardbound copy.

THE I CAN'T CHEW COOKBOOK: SAY...NUTS TO SOUP ONLY

Link: http://a.co/d/5VIU3nJ

Our next goal is to re-publish a 25th anniversary edition of "The I can't Chew Cookbook" using our interpretation of the book using perhaps modern artwork, perhaps interject our renditions of her recipes as well as add a generations' worth of evolution.

Can we ask a favor?

If you enjoyed this book, found it useful or otherwise then I'd really appreciate it if you would post a short review on Amazon. We do read all the reviews personally so that we can continually write what people are wanting.

If you'd like to leave a review then please visit the link below:

THE I CAN'T CHEW COOKBOOK: SAY...NUTS TO SOUP ONLY

Link: http://a.co/d/5VlU3nJ

Thanks for your support!

Jean Bly and Bly House Media